~~rn on or before th
~~ ~tamped below

GUIDES

THE BEAUTY INDUSTRY

REAL LIFE GUIDES

Practical guides for practical people

In this increasingly sophisticated world the need for manually skilled people to build our homes, cut our hair, fix our boilers, and make our cars go is greater than ever. As things progress, so the level of training and competence required of our skilled manual workers increases. In this series of career guides from Trotman, we look in detail at what it takes to train for, get into, and be successful at a wide spectrum of practical careers. The *Real Life Guides* aim to inform and inspire young people and adults alike by providing comprehensive yet hard-hitting and often blunt information about what it takes to succeed in these careers.

Other titles in the series are:

Real Life Guide: The Armed Forces
Real Life Guide: The Beauty Industry
Real Life Guide: Care
Real Life Guide: Carpentry and Cabinet-Making
Real Life Guide: Catering
Real Life Guide: Construction
Real Life Guide: Distribution and Logistics
Real Life Guide: Electrician
Real Life Guide: The Fire Service
Real Life Guide: Hairdressing
Real Life Guide: Plumbing
Real Life Guide: The Police Force
Real Life Guide: Retailing
Real Life Guide: Transport
Real Life Guide: Working Outdoors
Real Life Guide: Working with Animals and Wildlife
Real Life Guide: Working with Young People

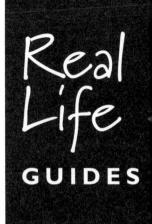

Real Life

GUIDES

THE BEAUTY INDUSTRY

Samantha Taylor

Second edition

Real Life Guide to the Beauty Industry
This second edition published in 2007 by Trotman
an imprint of Crimson Publishing,
Westminster House, Kew Road, Richmond, Surrey TW9 2ND
www.crimsonpublishing.co.uk

© Samantha Taylor 2007, 2004
First edition published 2004 by Trotman and Co Ltd

Author Samantha Taylor
Advertising Sarah Talbot, Advertising Sales Director

Designed by XAB

British Library Cataloguing in Publications Data
A catalogue record for this book is available from the British
Library

ISBN 978 1 84455 135 4

Typeset by Mac Style, Nafferton, East Yorkshire
Printed and bound in Great Britain by
Creative Print & Design, Wales

Real Life GUIDES

CONTENTS

About the author

Samantha Taylor has been involved in the beauty industry for 25 years as a therapist, educator and author. She first trained at Hastings College of Arts and Technology when beauty therapy wasn't as popular or admired as it is now. Throughout the years she has seen the many changes and improvements in the beauty field that make it what it is today. Currently she is a director of a national training company, course accreditor within schools and co-owner of a beauty salon. Her time is divided between teaching, assessing, verifying and writing books on all aspects of the industry for the education, careers and consumer market.

Acknowledgements

Thanks to two friends who are an integral part of my team of tutors, they are both reliable and flexible; industry specialists who are passionate about imparting their knowledge to the therapists of tomorrow. Louise and Jo, thanks for all your hard work and commitment!

Foreword

Can you help people feel good on the outside and the inside? If you think you can then perhaps you should try a career in beauty therapy. As a beauty therapist you need to create the right impression with your clients – professional, courteous and discreet – but still be personable.

Beauty is one of those careers where you can start at the bottom but can quickly work your way up. It's not uncommon for salon managers or owners, or for trainers in colleges to be in their twenties.

City & Guilds are delighted to be part of the Trotman *Real Life Guides* series to help raise your awareness of these vocational qualifications. If you're considering a career in beauty therapy, then you can get a City & Guilds qualification. Check out www.cityandguilds.com/myperfectjob to find your nearest college.

Introduction

A career in beauty therapy offers many different opportunities. You can do something you love, have fun, meet exciting people and even get the chance to travel, all whilst helping others feel good about themselves. From working in a salon, being your own boss, to cruising the seas – beauty can offer you all this and the chance to progress to management level with a top salary to match!

Exciting opportunities with good financial rewards in a flexible and fun environment are there for the right person.

Employment opportunities can range from working in health spas, hospitals and prisons to being a make-up artist on photographic shoots. You may eventually wish to share your knowledge and skills as an educator in a college or work on a beauty magazine as a writer. High demand for beauty therapists means that there is a vast range of opportunities within the industry and, although salaries can be low at the start, the chance to earn excellent wages is there for the right people.

Beauty therapy is a career that you can take with you, wherever your personal life leads you. There will always be someone who will want his or her legs waxed, feet pedicured and achy back massaged. It is no longer a luxury to have these treatments – they are all part of a busy person's lifestyle and maintenance. If you are first-rate at what you do, you will never be short of work.

The industry is worth an amazing £500 million so if you ask yourself 'will I get a job when I qualify'? The answer is yes; if you have had good training that has developed excellent skills, you will have the qualities required by employers and their many clients – there are currently 92 million client visits to beauty salons and spas a year.

Below are listed the latest statistics for the hair and beauty industry thanks to Habia (the Hairdressing and Beauty Industry Authority). All statistics are updated on a regular basis to ensure they are accurate and reflect the current state of the beauty industry in the UK.

	Beauty	**Hair**
Turnover	£500 million	£3.8 billion (including barbering)
Employees	35,000	31,000
Businesses	8,000	100,000
Client visits	92 million	340 million
Training	Awaiting update	100,000
Vacancies	6,550	37,000

Beauty therapy is not restrictive and gains strength from the wide range of talents, personalities, nationalities, abilities and ages that qualify. Although beauty salons can claim exemption from the Sex Discrimination Act and the vast majority of beauty and holistic therapists are female, the number of male therapists is rising – especially as it becomes more acceptable for men to take an interest in beauty treatments too!

In order to make informed decisions about a career in beauty you need to be able to find good-quality and accurate information about the industry – about the types of career options open to you, what you should expect to give to your career and what you can expect to get out of it, plus the sources of education and training that can help you get on. This guide is for anyone wanting to train, currently training or who is already qualified and wants to progress further. It details everything you need to know to help you make the right decisions. At the end of the book is a useful list of resources, which help you take your research further.

Job profiles

Mention the beauty industry and most people think of manicures, pedicures, facials and body waxing treatments that are offered in a high street salon. Of course these are an essential part of the industry but nowadays there is so much more to it than that. Available treatments and job opportunities are varied and fabulous – if you are interested in a career in beauty, the next step of your research starts here. The more unusual treatments on offer are holistic therapy, hydrotherapy (water-based treatments), electrical facial and body treatments, and spray tanning to name a few. The salon – and to a lesser extent the spa – certainly does form the heart and hub of the beauty profession, but there is a great deal more variety in the industry – both in terms of the range of jobs available and the location where these jobs are carried out, be it a cruise ship, hospital or department store.

In this chapter, we'll look at the full range of jobs available – the type of work they involve, the training they require, the pay and hours and what you can do now to get yourself into that particular area. Opposite, there's a diagram that will give you an overview of the opportunities available.

In every job, you cannot replace high-quality training on your path to success. The most widely recognised beauty-industry qualifications are known as National Vocational Qualifications (NVQs) or, in Scotland, the Scottish Vocational Qualifications (SVQs). There are four levels of NVQ, with level 1 the most basic. Each level is made up of a number of units, covering the various beauty techniques as well as other aspects of the work. There is a lot more

access to

BEAUTY THERAPY

Look at the career paths below and decide which one is right for you

HIGH STREET SALON

COLLEGE LEAVER
ASSISTANT BEAUTY THERAPIST
BEAUTY THERAPIST
SENIOR BEAUTY THERAPIST
ASSISTANT SALON MANAGER
SALON MANAGER OR SALON OWNER
GROUP SALON MANAGER

SALES CONSULTANT

COLLEGE LEAVER
COUNTER SALES ADVISER
COMPANY SALES REPRESENTATIVE/ PRODUCT TRAINER
COMPANY SALES MANAGER/ PRODUCT TRAINER
REGIONAL SALES MANAGER/ PRODUCT TRAINER
NATIONAL SALES MANAGER

SPA/HEALTH FARM

COLLEGE LEAVER
JUNIOR SPA THERAPIST
SPA THERAPIST
SENIOR SPA THERAPIST
ASSISTANT SPA MANAGER
SPA MANAGER

TEACHING

COLLEGE LEAVER
BEAUTY/SPA THERAPIST FOR APPROX 3–5 YEARS
PART-TIME COURSE TO QUALIFY INCL ASSESSOR AWARDS WHILST GAINING EXPERIENCE TEACHING OR;
PART-TIME COURSE FOR CERTIFICATE IN EDUCATION INCL ASSESSOR AWARDS WHILST GAINING EXPERIENCE TEACHING
LECTURER/ASSESSOR – FE, PRIVATE OR WORK-BASED
INTERNAL VERIFIER/EXAMINER/ EXTERNAL VERIFIER

Or you may instead choose to follow a career in make-up or nail technology if you choose these options within your NVQ

*Further and Adult Education Teachers Certificate

about NVQs and SVQs, as well as other qualifications, in the Training chapter.

BEAUTY CONSULTANT

As a beauty consultant you would help your customers to choose the right beauty products for their lifestyle, to make the most of their personal appearance. Most beauty consultants work on the cosmetic counters in department stores or large pharmacies. However there are opportunities at airports, large hotels and cruise liners. Your job would involve spending time with customers, analysing clients' skin, carrying out makeovers and giving skincare and make-up lessons. You will need to understand skin type, face shape and colouring, and know which products will be most effective and best suit your customer's colouring, lifestyle and age. You need to keep up to date with new skincare products, perfumes and make-up.

To do this work you should have a smart appearance and be well groomed, have excellent interpersonal skills and be good at selling and arranging displays.

To do this work you should have a smart appearance and be well groomed, have excellent interpersonal skills and be good at selling and arranging displays. You will also need to have an outgoing and friendly personality as well as excellent communication skills.

Training

Although you do not have to have specific qualifications to become a beauty consultant, you will still need a good standard of general education with good literacy and numeracy skills. You will probably do on-the-job training run by the company you work for, however there are some excellent qualifications if you wish to study for a consultancy qualification. These can be attended on a full- or part-time basis at college.

- VTCT (Vocational Training Charitable Trust) Certificate in Beauty Consultancy
- VTCT Certificate in Cosmetic Make-up
- City & Guilds level 2 Certificate and Diploma in Beauty Consultancy
- BTEC level 2 Certificate and Diploma in Retail Beauty Consultancy
- ITEC qualifications.

Training offered by a product company will not usually result in a recognised qualification.

Training offered by a product company will not usually result in a recognised qualification, such as those listed above, and therefore will not lead to a career in beauty therapy. So be sure that you know what your future aims are.

Pay and hours

You'll work around 37–40 hours per week and you will be expected to work at weekends. Starting salaries could be around £10,000 a year. Experienced consultants may earn up to and over £19,000. Salaries will rise according to experience, and many companies offer incentives such as staff discounts and commission on sales. Consultants are expected to meet sales targets so the job may be quite pressurised.

The good
Seeing customers walk out holding their head up high after you've given them a makeover or sold them some fantastic products can be a thrill. It is especially satisfying to see clients return to you time after time because they know that you can give sound advice and recognise their type of skin and individual needs.

The bad
Being on your feet all day! Occasionally you may have a very demanding client, and having to ensure that your appearance remains immaculate all day, no matter how tired or busy you are, can be hard work. You must appear unflappable, capable and efficient with a ready smile and a polite manner, whatever!

Advice for students
Get a Saturday job behind the counter in a department store or large pharmacy so that you get a feel of the job and what it's all about – and whether you can stand on your feet all day with a smile on your face!

SALON BEAUTY SPECIALIST/THERAPIST

Becoming a beauty specialist (otherwise known as a beautician) is generally the first step towards being a beauty therapist and can be achieved in one year on a full-time basis, with the award of an NVQ level 2 or equivalent. Some learners only want to achieve this level, deciding to concentrate on skincare, nail treatments, make-up, eye treatments and wax depilation rather than the additional skills offered at NVQ level 3. Beauty therapists, who carry out procedures such as electrolysis and body treatments are qualified to NVQ level 3 or equivalent.

A salon therapist will be expected to carry out a variety of treatments throughout the day. It is vital that booking times are kept to so that clients are not kept waiting in reception. Salons can be hectic, so you need a **calm, efficient manner** to deal with the high volume of clients you will deal with in just one day. In an eight-hour day you could carry out treatments on more than 20 clients! Spa and holistic therapists will carry out a variety of massage and spa treatments in a relaxing and therapeutic environment, such as a health farm, spa or therapy centre.

Training

There is a wide range of options, but typically a two-year course full time at college will result in an NVQ level 3. Other options are combined college and workplace training such as the Apprenticeship schemes (see Chapter 7) or shorter courses at private colleges. You may wish to start as an assistant or junior therapist by doing qualifications such as NVQ level 1 in Beauty Therapy.

Funding for apprenticeships is available for 16–24 year olds and some over-25s. To find out more, visit www.apprenticeships.org.uk.

Once qualified at NVQ level 3 as a beauty therapist, you could decide to:

- specialise in one of the treatments such as electrolysis or body work
- train to qualify in other areas of beauty and complementary therapies
- progress to level 4 for a career in beauty management
- City & Guilds NVQ levels 1, 2 and 3 in Beauty Therapy
- Edexcel NVQ level 1, 2 and 3 in Beauty Therapy
- Edexcel National Certificate/Diploma in Beauty Therapy Sciences
- VTCT Diploma in Beauty Therapy.

Pay and hours

Pay may be low to start with, but for experienced therapists who bring in a lot of money for the business the potential to earn a substantial wage is there, particularly if you are paid commission on top. See Chapter 4 for more about incomes.

You're never bored in a busy salon because of the wide range of treatments you cover in one day.

Therapists normally work a five-day week but some salons operate on six and seven days. If your salon is like this you will be expected to work a rota system whereby every member of staff takes a turn to work the unsocial hours, including late opening in the evenings. You will still be entitled to a fixed day off per week though, and your hours should not exceed employment guidelines.

The good

You're never bored in a busy salon because of the wide range of treatments you cover in one day. Each client and each treatment are always different. You also get to work with and meet many different people.

The bad

At times you may be extremely busy, with aching legs and feet, and no time for even so much as a cup of tea. That's when you feel anything but calm. Imagine it – a client has turned up late and made you get behind with your other clients; the phone is ringing; the receptionist is at lunch; and behind your smile and calm exterior you could happily scream! Remember, though, the good does outweigh the bad!

> **DID YOU KNOW?**
>
> There are approximately 8,000 beauty salons in the UK.

Advice for students

After college, gain employment and experience in a salon that employs quite a few other staff, so that you learn from them. Try to stay in your first job for at least a year, as anything less doesn't look great on your CV. A year in one place will teach you a great deal about the industry. Accept any offer of training from your employer and look out for short courses in order to update and extend your skills.

NAIL TECHNICIAN

Nail technicians use creativity and skill to improve the appearance and condition of clients' nails. They will carry out manicures and pedicures, as well as applying and maintaining nail extensions, and decorating the nails using nail art techniques such as paint, glitter, gem and jewellery application, airbrushing and stencilling. Nail technicians must have good communication skills, they will discuss the type of nail treatment wanted, check for any conditions that will affect treatment and give aftercare and retail advice to clients. Technicians need to work quickly and efficiently with great attention to detail and be highly organised and tidy.

Hygiene, health and safety are very important parts of the job because the chemicals used are flammable or can irritate and therefore need to be stored correctly. Tools must also be sterilised properly to prevent infection or fungal growth to the natural nail underneath.

Training

NVQ levels 2 and 3 now offer training routes for nail technicians, covering the essential knowledge and practical assessments needed to gain access to the industry. Awarding bodies are listed in Chapter 9 along with details of their websites, where all courses can be viewed.

Suitable courses are:

- NVQ/SVQ level 2 in Nail Services (for junior nail technicians)
- NVQ/SVQ level 3 in Nail Services (for senior/salon nail technicians).

Pay and hours

A newly qualified nail technician can expect the **national minimum wage** particularly if working in a salon or nail bar. Brilliant money is out there for top technicians, who are in demand for education, session work, magazine and photographic work. A highly experienced self-employed nail technician can earn in excess of £25,000, particularly when in demand for media work or is the owner of a nail bar.

Hours will tend to be fairly set if working in a salon, but self-employed work can be unsociable with long hours.

The good
There is the pleasure of seeing clients leave the salon with renewed confidence as they look down at their beautiful nails. If you are really successful, the job could take you all over the world, with supermodels or celebrity clients. There is also the opportunity to pass on your expertise by training new nail technicians.

The bad
Sitting for long periods of time leant over a nail station can wreak havoc on your back and neck. Also the smells of the nail products can be very strong and overpowering. Good posture and ventilation are crucial.

Advice for students
After training, shadow an experienced nail technician for a couple of months, even if you don't get paid! This grounding will teach you so much more about the clients, high standards and speed and accuracy needed to get on in the business. Enter competitions if you can (see Chapter 9 – 'Further Information'). If you win or get placed, this will give you free publicity for your skills and put your name and face on the industry map.

MOBILE BEAUTY THERAPIST
Once you have trained and gained some salon experience, you may decide to branch out on your own. Mobile treatments require a lot of organisation, but are worth doing if you need to work around family commitments. If you are also wary of paying rent and the large overheads that owning your own salon brings, then this is the way to go as long as you don't mind carrying around equipment from house to house. An important fact to remember is that you could end up covering unnecessary miles if you

don't work out your routes and **organise yourself** to work within a certain area for a particular day or period of time. The range of clients is wide, but quite a large proportion of business can come from care homes and hospitals, parents at home with small children and the disabled and elderly. So ensure that you target this large client group with your advertising methods. Alternatively you could set up a home practice if you prefer a base to work from.

Training
The usual recognised beauty therapy training – a minimum of NVQ/SVQ level 2 – is needed.

Pay and hours
The pay really depends on you. If you are very businesslike with your scheduling, travel arrangements and appointment bookings, you can successfully earn a very good salary. Remember, though, the best advertising is word of mouth, so keep those clients happy!

The hours, too, can vary – remember that mobile therapists can do a lot of their work in the evenings when people have finished work and want a relaxing evening at home having a massage. The popular thing nowadays is pamper parties where a hostess arranges for a few friends to come around and have treatments by a beauty therapist.

The good
The overheads are low – just the running of your vehicle (plus electricity if home-based), as well as product costs. It is essential that you have insurance and council registration so that you are fully-covered. You are also in control of your working hours and what you do with them.

The bad
It can be lonely working on your own, especially when you are faced with a problem or important decision and there's no one with you to give advice. It can also involve lots of driving around and carrying heavy equipment in all weathers. There is also the less pleasant aspect of working at home after normal working hours because you will need to do your bookkeeping and accounts, stock checking and ordering, equipment cleaning and maintenance and laundry.

Advice for students
Don't expect to be able to work alone straight from college, you need the experience of salon work. If you eventually decide to go mobile, then check out the area – is it needed? If you know someone in a different area that does mobile treatments, ask for their advice. Finally, speak to a small-business adviser and get as much information about running your own business as you can. Have a separate telephone number apart from your home one, otherwise you will find yourself on call 24 hours a day – a mobile number for business is the best solution.

Be strict about your treatment time. Tell clients how long you expect the treatment to take and that you will need to leave by a certain time. Clients answering telephone calls and seeing to the family will eat into your time and end up costing you money and making you late for your next appointment. Choose your products and equipment carefully – the equipment must be hard-wearing and the products (such as wax) where possible should be water-based to facilitate cleaning if spilt.

WORKING ON CRUISE LINERS

Jobs in this field are available for beauty therapists, massage therapists and nail technicians. You will be working in a top-class establishment, albeit on the waves. You will be expected to get on with everyone, both the 1,000–3,000 passengers and the 500–1,500 crew members. So the **ability to work in a team** is essential. Each contract is for approximately eight months, and during this time you will share an extremely small cabin with another spa team member. You are required to be **physically and emotionally healthy**. You must have a medical before joining ship.

DID YOU KNOW?

You may be a long distance from family but keeping in touch is easy, most ships have internet cafes, satellite phones and postal services as well as payphones in ports where the ship will dock 3–4 times a week.

With luxury and top class entertainment on board and routes to fantastic destinations the cruise industry is geared up for the masses and is one of the fastest growing sectors of the travel industry. It is no longer for the rich and privileged few.

Cruise staff work hard, the expectations of passengers and management is high. The life is fast paced, hours long and accommodation cramped – you don't go home at the end of a hard day!

Training

Beauty therapists must be qualified to level 3 standard with one of the recognised awarding bodies. Facial and body massage, including electrical face and body treatments, is essential.

Massage therapists must be qualified in Swedish massage with a recognised qualification. Additional qualifications in therapies such as shiatsu, reflexology, reiki, sports massage and aromatherapy are a great advantage.

Nail technicians must be qualified with good industrial experience in all nail-enhancement systems (for example gel and acrylic). They also need to be qualified in manicure and pedicure. An NVQ level 2 and 3 or recognised nail technician course is expected.

Pay and hours
Hours can be long, and you will be expected to do shift work so that flexible working patterns can be arranged to cover evening work. The pay depends on your position on board and your experience. However, most of your earnings will come from commission. Tips from passengers can seriously increase your earnings.

The good
Career prospects and opportunities for promotion within the company are good. There will be the chance to see places around the world as you will get some time off at ports of call.

The bad
Sharing what is little more than a cupboard as a bedroom can be taxing. On board ship you are never off-duty. The fast-paced life can be hectic and stressful, as is being away from home for such a long period of time. Homesickness and seasickness are both very possible!

Advice for students
If this is a longer-term goal, you should first complete your beauty-therapy training and go into industry for a couple of

years in order to develop a mature outlook and treatment experience. During this time, try to expand your skills with further training in order to give yourself a head start above other job candidates. Start applying to cruise-liner companies six months before you want to start so that you have time to attend interviews and have medicals. Interviews are ongoing and UK-wide, visit www.steinerleisure.com to find out about jobs available.

INFLIGHT BEAUTY THERAPIST

This is physically demanding work, as you will be on your feet constantly during flights. You must be friendly, approachable and polite at all times. You must be technically excellent because the treatments are carried out on First Class passengers who expect the best. Even after a long-haul flight **your grooming must be immaculate**. You will fly from Heathrow. Excellent health is essential as is a preliminary training course. You must be a minimum of 18 years of age, 5' 2" minimum in height, fluent in English and a holder of a European Union passport, as well as having salon experience of at least one year.

The beauty treatments are free in Upper Class (business class) and are now available on all return flights leaving Heathrow. The different types of therapies include 'Back in the Clouds', 'Hands – Zone Therapy', and 'Hot Hands'.

Your duties will also include taking responsibility for the safety of customers and fellow crew for the duration of the flight. The work is physically demanding and you will often work through the night, so you must be in excellent health. Currently these jobs are only available on Virgin Atlantic but other airlines may start offering this service to passengers, so it is worth doing some research.

Training

You'll need a minimum of three GCSE passes (or equivalent) plus you must be fully qualified in all aspects of beauty therapy, holding one of the following qualifications (or their equivalent) BTEC HND, CIBTAC/C&G/VTCT NVQ level 2 plus the body massage unit at level 3 as a minimum. Qualifications in Indian head massage and aromatherapy are an advantage but not essential.

Pay and hours

Airlines offer a good basic salary package, which includes flight allowances and commission payments. Holiday is 28 days per year. After complying with certain criteria, you will also be offered concessionary travel, private medical insurance and pension schemes.

The good

You'll have global travel opportunities and the chance to meet interesting people.

The bad

There will be long tiring flights and some demanding passengers, and you will have to take your turn to work bank holidays, including Christmas. Remember the unsociable hours can disrupt your social life.

Advice for students

Go into industry, gain experience and then apply to an airline through its website. Even if not selected, keep trying. Competition is tough – so you may find that the more experience you gain the more chance you have of getting in, as the airline beauty industry is expanding all the time.

SALON OWNER

For this profile, we will assume that you are a qualified beauty therapist, simply because you would not have the skills, understanding and background knowledge to run your own beauty salon and a team of staff – unless you employed a beauty therapist as the day-to-day manager.

Competition between salons can be fierce, but if yours is well run, with quality treatments being carried out, you can succeed. As owner, you would be expected to carry out treatments, organise staff rotas, carry out payroll paperwork and wages, complete monthly and end-of-year accounts, order stock, stocktake, interview and employ new staff, arrange PR and advertising and much more. Your day would start before the staff arrive and finish after they have gone home. Being your own boss is not necessarily the best option; it can be mentally and physically exhausting and can try your patience at the best of times.

Training

Level 3 Beauty Therapy or equivalent is the basic level required, while a management qualification is a definite advantage.

Pay and hours

This can vary enormously, depending on how busy the salon is, where the business is situated, how many staff you need to pay and so on. It is best to set yourself a small salary, and at the year end see what profit has been made, what equipment needs to be replaced, which staff need pay rises and what decoration and alterations need doing before finally deciding whether to increase your salary.

Being your own boss is not necessarily the best option; it can be mentally and physically exhausting and can try your patience at the best of times.

The good
You will hopefully get a great sense of satisfaction from what you have achieved, especially if your business is thriving and you have a sense of pride in what you do.

The bad
Long hours, sorting out staff problems or disagreements and managing paperwork and administration are just a few of the headaches. Another is the worry when the business hits a slow period of the year and bookings fall.

Advice for students
Don't even think about setting up your own business until you have had a few jobs and experienced the good and not so good ways that salons are run. Take it all in, hone your skills and learn as much as you can about the non-treatment side of beauty therapy. Undertake a management course whilst working in a salon.

ELECTROLYSIST

This job involves treating unwanted hair growth by inserting a fine sterile needle into the hair follicle and passing a mild, controlled electrical current through it to the root of the hair. This cauterises the hair-production area, which enables the hair to be lifted out by forceps (electrolysis tweezers). This is a gradual weakening process that destroys the hair over a number of treatments.

You must have **excellent interpersonal skills** as the treatment can be very intimate, involving close work and knowledge of the client's medical history. Clients are often very self-conscious of their hair growth and need to be put at ease from the start. Comprehensive knowledge of the skin and hair and of health and safety are essential, as is **good eyesight** and **steady hands**.

Training

You can follow the NVQ level 3 general route; choose the epilation unit as an additional option if taking an alternative level 3 route (for example Spa or Nail Services) or take another appropriate examination course. Awarding bodies such as VTCT, City & Guilds, Edexcel and ITEC offer suitable courses. Membership of the British Association of Electrolysists (see Chapter 9 for contact details) is subject to an additional examination as it expects standards to be very high.

Pay and hours

Pay is in line with salon wages for the level of experience unless you are self-employed. Working as an electrolysist on a mobile basis is not particularly financially viable as many of the sessions are short, as little as ten minutes at a time. It is far better to work from a base such as home or as a chair-renter. Hours are quite standard unless self-employed, in which case you will be expected to carry out some evening work.

The good

The emotional boost a client gets from seeing unwanted hair disappearing is enormous. It gives the therapist a huge boost, too, to see how they have helped a client who may have been lacking in self-esteem and social confidence.

The bad
Such close work involving accuracy and concentration can affect the eyes over a period of time. This may just be eyestrain or occasional headaches. If good posture is not maintained, back and neck problems can occur.

It gives the therapist a huge boost to see how they have helped a client who may have been lacking in self-esteem and social confidence.

Advice for students
Develop your skills in the workplace first, and then apply for membership to the British Association of Electrolysists. The association gives out names of its members to potential clients looking for practitioners in their area, keeps you informed of new developments and holds seminars for professional development.

DID YOU KNOW?

British beauty therapy is recognised as the best in the world.

CAMOUFLAGE MAKE-UP SPECIALIST
In this job, you will cover birthmarks, scars, accident injuries and burns using corrective make-up techniques and specialist make-up. The job could be freelance, going where the work takes you. A lot of the work could be hospital-based in special units.

Training
This subject is a unit within level 3 Beauty Therapy courses. This will provide you with the necessary background knowledge of the skin and anatomy as well as the basics of make-up before you move into more specialised and sensitive topics.

Pay and hours
If freelance, pay and hours could vary greatly as you will be doing your own costings. If employed, however, they will follow the requirements of the national minimum wage as a minimum.

The good
You will get enormous job satisfaction from seeing people cosmetically improved where once they had disfiguring marks that caused them great distress and embarrassment.

The bad
Some disfigurements can be distressful to the onlooker. You need to remember that it's just visual and your job is to improve the appearance of it for the client.

Advice for students
Contact the National Health Service (NHS) and private hospitals for information about remedial camouflage. They will be able to advise you as to the best way to go. Usually you can't go wrong if you shadow an experienced person. This will give you both experience and contacts.

SALES REPRESENTATIVE
A sales representative is employed by a product, equipment or cosmetic company to sell its goods to salons and spas

nationally or regionally. The job involves a lot of travelling around, meeting prospective suppliers and answering their queries. You must be completely knowledgeable about the product that you are promoting and sincerely believe in it yourself. Your attitude must be **professional, efficient** and **organised**. There will also be an element of paperwork, such as appointment scheduling, record-keeping and sales data.

Training
A beauty therapy or consultancy background is ideal so that you have the essential knowledge of the industry and salon/spa requirements for business success. Once you have experience as a therapist or consultant, knowledge in various brands will also stand you in good stead. For example, if you undertook extra training in a range of skincare brands you would be at an advantage if a job were advertised for the particular brand you had trained in.

Pay and hours
These can vary, but sales representatives are usually offered a yearly salary with commission on sales. A company car and other benefits such as discounts and healthcare can also be offered.

The good
Being independent is a plus. You get to make your own appointments, research your area and follow up contacts which, when good, can lead to a big sale or a company account on the books.

The bad
On a bad day, you could be travelling around all day without anyone being interested in taking on the product.

Advice for students
Get experience as a beauty consultant or beauty/spa therapist and, whilst working, undertake continuous development in new/existing treatments and products so that you are ready for when the particular company you are interested in is recruiting.

SPORTS MASSAGE THERAPIST
The job involves massage and manipulation of the muscles and joints. The massage itself is much deeper and more intense than a Swedish massage and **you need a strong physique and hands**, as the work is very physically demanding. Sports massage is a special form of massage and is typically used before, during and after athletic events. The purpose of the massage is to prepare the athlete for peak performance, to drain away fatigue, to relieve swelling, to reduce muscle tension, to promote flexibility and to prevent injuries. Sports massage can help prevent those niggling injuries that so often get in the way of performance and achievement, whether a person is an athlete or a once-a-week jogger.

Training
You will need to achieve a qualification in anatomy, physiology and body massage before advancing to a sports massage qualification from a recognised awarding body. Contact the Federation of Holistic Therapists ((FHT) www.fht.org.uk) for further guidance.

Pay and hours

Sports massage is usually offered in health clubs and fitness centres or as a freelance service and occasionally in hospitals. If you're lucky, you can be assigned to work for a sports team as their sports massage therapist. If you have a good reputation, then you can expect to charge a good hourly rate that takes into account your expertise. There may be a lot of weekend work, especially if you are part of a sports team.

DID YOU KNOW?

There are other types of massage — Indian head massage, baby massage and Swedish body massage — why not research them to find out more.

The good

Job satisfaction may come from alleviating a person's pain and discomfort or from treating muscles to keep them fit and healthy.

The bad

This is a very strenuous job that can cause aches and pains in you if you don't maintain correct posture. Freelancing also involves a lot of driving around to clients, sometimes at very unsociable hours. You go where and when you are needed.

Advice for students

Whilst training, volunteer your services to a local team at the weekend so that you can practise your sports massage skills. If they already have a qualified person, then ask if you can shadow them. You will pick up lots of good techniques and advice. Alternatively ask a local health club, fitness centre or physiotherapy department in a hospital if you can do work experience for them.

MAKE-UP ARTIST

Theatrical make-up involves applying period and costume make-up for plays and productions and very often very elaborate fantasy make-up. Just think of the musical *Lion King*. Media involves making up actors, celebrities, models and presenters, along with carrying out high-fashion make-up for magazine work, photographic shoots and platform/runway shows. Television and film make-up involves much of the above plus designing and making prosthetics. Prosthetics are false facial and body features that change the appearance of an actor. It all sounds very glamorous but be prepared to work very long hours on your feet.

You can specialise in theatrical, media or television and film make-up, but if you have a wealth of experience behind you, you could become an all-rounder. There are general differences between the areas, but a lot of the skills tend to overlap at times.

Creativity is essential, as is tact and patience, as you will be working within a demanding industry.

A large part of make-up artistry involves hair, as wigs, hairpieces, beards and moustaches are also used, so a hairdressing qualification would give you a distinct advantage. Many employers in this area of the industry will not employ you without one. You will certainly also need a **good sense of colour**, balance and design. **Creativity is essential**, as is **tact** and **patience**, as you will be working within a demanding industry. You must be able to work under pressure and have good communication skills.

Training

The starting point is qualifications in beauty and hairdressing, especially as NVQ Beauty now offers the make-up route. Suitable courses are:

- BTEC National Certificate/Diploma in Production Arts (Make-up)
- VTCT level 3 Diploma in Theatre and Media Make-up
- ITEC level 3 Diploma in Fashion, Theatre and Media Make-up
- HNCs/HNDs in Media Make-up.

You would then need to take a course in TV and film make-up or be an apprentice to a freelance make-up artist so that you can learn the trade first hand. Film and Television Freelance Training ((FT2) www.FT2.org.uk) runs a two-year apprenticeship-style New Entrant Technical Training Scheme for make-up and hair assistants. Places are strictly limited and the selection process is tough. In addition Skillset offer subsidised courses. You must be:

- aged 18 or over
- minimum qualification NVQ/SVQ level 2 in Hairdressing and Beauty Therapy
- prepared to live in London during training.

Pay and hours

Hours can vary greatly. You need to take the work as it comes because if you freelance you may have long periods without assignments. The pay can be excellent particularly if you're in demand. You will be working for a daily fee, which usually starts at the industry minimum of £100 per day for a junior make-up/hair assistant; £150 for a make-up designer/prosthetics. Higher rates apply for commercials, which can be in excess of £500 per day for experienced artists. Fashion and editorial work ranges from £200 to £2,000 per day. Top make-up artists for fashion shows regularly earn over £3,000 per day. (Rates courtesy of: Producers Alliance for Cinema and Television (PACT), Broadcasting Entertainment Cinematographic and Theatre Union (BECTU).)

The good
There's the possibility of extensive travel to exotic places, meeting famous people, seeing your work on the big screen, and seeing your name credited in magazines, shows and television. Working on such a wide variety of projects and assignments makes it hard to get bored.

The bad
The job can involve a lot of standing around and waiting, especially in the TV and film industry. You'll be under pressure to work to strict timescales and you will need to fit in around other people. A lot of the people that you make up are very demanding and can test your patience.

Advice for Students
GCSEs in subjects such as art, history and human anatomy would be very helpful. Be prepared to work unpaid in amateur dramatics and local theatre companies to gain experience and build up a portfolio to show prospective employees.

HOLISTIC THERAPIST
In this job, you might specialise in Indian head massage, aromatherapy, reflexology, hot stones, thermal auricular (ear

candling) therapy, reiki, crystal and colour therapy or even be qualified to offer them all.

Aromatherapy uses blends of essential oils that have been extracted from flowers, trees, spices, fruit or herbs. The oils have healing and relaxing properties and can be applied by massage, baths, compresses and inhalations. Aromatherapy is also used in hospitals to boost ill patients.

DID YOU KNOW?

Male beauty is big business! The male grooming market was valued at £685 million in 2004 and is expected to be worth £821 million by 2009.

Indian head massage is based on traditional Indian techniques that use a variety of massage movements. It is a unique and versatile treatment involving massage of the scalp, neck and shoulders to induce relaxation and a feeling of well-being.

Reflexology uses specialised massage techniques on the soles of the feet. The soles represent a mirror image or map of the body, and by massaging parts of the feet you can unblock energy pathways and alleviate minor ailments in the body. It is best used as a preventative measure against more serious ailments.

Can you find out more about hot stones and ear candling?

Training
There are no specific entry requirements to train as a holistic therapist. However, some courses expect you to have a basic massage qualification first. You will also be expected

to learn about the anatomy and physiology of the body. This may be a separate course that runs alongside the practical part, or it may be built into the qualification, depending on the award that you are studying for. There are many courses available, both private and state-run, but make sure that if you study privately the course is a recognised and endorsed qualification from a well-known awarding body or you will not be able to obtain insurance. VTCT offer many courses for holistic therapy as detailed below.

- Level 1 Certificate in Introduction to Therapies (Holistic)
- Level 2 Certificate in Holistic Therapies
- Level 2 Certificate in Thermal Auricular Therapy
- Level 3 Diploma in Aromatherapy
- Level 3 Diploma in Holistic Consultation Techniques
- Level 3 Diploma in Holistic Therapies
- Level 3 Diploma in Reflexology
- Level 3 Diploma for Reiki Practitioners

Pay and hours
If you are mobile, then the hours you work are your choice, but because of the popularity of holistic treatments you could be in great demand. The cost of the treatment to the client can range from £20 to £40. The nature of holistic therapies demands that the treatment be carried out in a calm and stress-free manner and environment, so rushing from one client to the next is not going to work. In a salon or spa you can expect to earn the minimum wage upwards, depending on your experience and position.

The good
The satisfaction comes from seeing how you can turn a wound-up, stressed-out client into a relaxed, chilled-out person before they leave. High levels of stress are causing

illness and even shortening our lives, so feeling that you have played a part in cutting down that stress can give you an enormous sense of satisfaction.

The bad
Holistic therapy is a very giving treatment and can be very emotionally draining, especially if you are carrying out six holistic treatments in one day.

Advice for students
Get experience in the industry first – as a masseur or beauty therapist – to gain experience with clients. Holistic therapists need a very mature attitude and a high level of life experience in order to be in a position to offer these type of treatments successfully and for a client to feel at ease with them.

BEAUTY WRITER
This could take the form of a staff writer on a health and beauty magazine, a freelance journalist specialising in beauty or an author of educational books and materials for a publisher. You must be prepared to work to tight deadlines. It can be very interesting work because you get the low-down on all the new products, techniques and training.

You need a **good knowledge of the English language** and good word-processing and keyboard skills. Be prepared to carry out extensive research to ensure that you write accurate and up-to-date material. You need to have a **determined personality** in order to be able to take the rejection of material returned or refused. Don't give up!

Training

A good background in beauty therapy is a distinct advantage, otherwise your background knowledge would have to rely completely on research instead of a combination of that and first hand experience. A course in writing and journalism is advisable, as is a GCSE in English.

Pay and hours

This varies enormously depending on whether you are writing a book or just a column in a magazine. If you write books and are paid on a royalty basis, the industry average is 10% of net receipt (sales), or you could be paid a one-off fee for the book instead. For information on magazine and periodical rates, *The Writer's Handbook* edited by Barry Turner is a good guide as it also lists all the magazines and newspapers in the UK and Europe. Hours can be long if you are working to a deadline.

The good

You may like working under your own steam and being able to do some writing jobs around other commitments. Seeing your writing actually in print gives you a great sense of satisfaction.

The bad

There's the tight, sore muscles in the neck and shoulders from being sat at a computer for so many hours, and sometimes you have to burn the midnight oil to get work finished. Additional hazards are the possible repetitive strain injury from using the keyboard and eyestrain from staring at a computer screen for long periods of time. It is also unusual to earn enough just writing; you will usually combine this with another job.

Advice for students

Visit publishers' and magazine houses' websites to check out their jobs and submission advice. Check out *The Writer's Handbook* for companies that accept samples of your writing. Alternatively, ask to do work experience on a magazine so that you get some useful contacts as well as seeing how the system works. For training in magazine journalism, visit the website of the Periodicals Training Council at www.ppa.co.uk. Membership bodies include the Writers' Guild of Great Britain (www.writersguild.org.uk) and The Society of Authors (www.societyofauthors.net).

DID YOU KNOW?

Currently there are about 500 approved training providers for hair and beauty offering beauty qualifications in the UK alone.

LECTURER/TRAINER

You can work as a company/product trainer or get a part-time or full-time job in a private or further education (FE) college. The groups of students in an FE college can vary in size from one to 18, but the important thing is that you must have the ability to impart information in a clear, accurate and interesting way. Your methods must be **well planned** and **organised**. You also need a firm but fair hand in order to maintain a professional level of conduct in teaching salons where there are actual paying clients.

Training

You will have completed your basic training and achieved NVQ/SVQ level 3 in Beauty Therapy. After gaining a few years' experience you then need to attend a part-time course at college to gain the City & Guilds Certification in Further Education Teaching, which gives you the basic grounding in how to teach students, plan your lessons and organise your class. You may then decide to progress to a teaching degree such as a Post Graduate Certificate in Education (PGCE) or a Certificate in Education (Cert Ed). You will be expected to carry out teaching practice during your training and will be assessed on your competence in teaching students. When training for a teaching qualification, you will also be expected to gain an assessor award, without which you will not be able to assess students.

Pay and hours
A full-time salary in an FE college rises with experience – the range is from approximately £16,000 to £30,000. Private colleges will have their own salary scale, and if you are a part-time lecturer you will be paid hourly.

The good
Getting groups of students through their qualification can give you a real kick – seeing how they have developed from day one until they graduate, and feeling that you had a lot to do with their achievements.

The bad
There's lots of preparation, marking and paperwork, much of which you will have to take home to complete. Although the holidays may seem long, it is extremely rare for you not to have to take work home with you during these breaks. Then there's dealing with the odd difficult learner who challenges your authority and expertise.

Advice for students
You will need to gain a few years experience in the industry before you even think about teaching. Approach a few

educational establishments to sound out their recruitment methods – as always, a bit of shadowing does no harm for picking up tips and contacts.

MAKING YOUR MIND UP

You should now have a good idea of the wealth of opportunities that exist in the beauty industry. Perhaps you've already decided which direction you would like to go in – you might always have known! – but if you're still unsure, you may find it useful to visit two government careers websites – www.connexions-direct.com and www.educationuk.org. Both sites are excellent sources of careers advice for the student wishing to pursue a career.

Now you've got another choice to make – where are you going to get that all-important training?

2

How to get in and on

By now you should have more of an idea whether a career in beauty is for you. There is the right job and training for everyone interested in the beauty industry. The most difficult choice is where and how to train and deciding on which career path to take. In this chapter, you'll find some more about how to track down the right course for you. On page 41, there's an easy-to-follow flow chart showing the whole process of interviewing and enrolling for a course. There's also more about training in Chapter 7.

GENERAL TRAINING

In every job, you cannot replace high-quality training on your path to success. The jobs showcased in Chapter 1 give a brief idea of qualifications required but this will be covered in more depth in Chapter 7.

CHOOSING A GOOD TRAINING CENTRE

With a wide range of beauty therapy courses available and many different training centres to choose from, where do you start? When looking at a college prospectus or phoning for information on a training centre, the Hairdressing and Beauty Industry Authority (Habia) advises prospective students to investigate:

● the number of students on the course and the staff/student ratio

- the length of the course and whether it's full or part time
- whether it's free and whether you would be eligible for a grant
- whether you qualify for tax relief on the training fee or a Career Development Loan, if you are paying
- whether the course leads to an NVQ/SVQ in Hairdressing or Beauty Therapy or any other approved qualification in the National Qualification Framework
- what level the course will reach
- how many students were on the course last year, how many achieved the required level and how many of them got jobs
- whether you can complete the course unit by unit, returning at a convenient time to complete any outstanding units
- what will be expected of you in terms of daily/weekly/ monthly assessments and exams
- how much equipment is provided and how much additional equipment will cost
- whether you can have a look around the college or training centre and meet for a chat with the trainers and current students
- the enrolment procedure – can you enrol at any time or are there set dates?
- whether you will be given a placement in a local salon to develop your skills, or be expected to find one yourself
- what options for training routes are available
- whether the centre has a quality award from an external organisation, such as a Chartermark or National Training Award.

You'll need to weigh up the advantages and disadvantages of what's available and decide on the training option that suits your circumstances best. Remember, your college entrance interview is a chance for you to find out more about the course just as much as it is a chance for them to find out about you! Be prepared to ask questions, such as whether there are grants available or whether there's childcare. This type of information may well help you in your decision-making. Below, we'll look at some of the issues listed above in a bit more detail.

PART TIME OR FULL TIME?

Being a full-time student is not the only way to learn. If you're working, unemployed or have family commitments, you can still study and get qualifications. Part-time and home study requires a lot of self-discipline though, especially when you need to fit it around the demands of your home and work life. But if you've got the determination, you can do it.

Being a full-time student is not the only way to learn. If you're working, unemployed or have family commitments, you can still study and get qualifications.

Choosing whether to study part or full time is crucial because rules about whether you pay and how much you pay for a course depend on this. It may also affect the kind of support you get for living expenses. Think things through carefully. Some of your options are listed below.

ENTRY TO COLLEGE

TELEPHONE OR CALL IN
FOR A PROSPECTUS

CHOOSE A COURSE

COMPLETE THE APPLICATION FORM

ATTEND A COURSE INTERVIEW AND COLLEGE VISIT

- Immaculate appearance and positive attitude
- Take Record of Achievement to be looked through and or references if adult learner
- Questions prepared about the course etc
- Will be given information on course fees and financial help

LETTER OF ACCEPTANCE

Should detail:
- date of enrolment
- place and time of enrolment
- what to bring

ENROLMENT

- Enrolment paperwork completed
- Course start date and times given
- Some colleges arrange facility for kit and uniform purchase at this
- May be given recommended book reading list

START OF TERM

Free courses
Full-time students, aged 16–19 years old, who study at a publicly-funded school or college don't have to pay tuition fees. If you claim a benefit, or rely on somebody who claims a benefit, you may get your fees paid in full or in part.

Getting a job
If you want to get a job after Year 11, it's important to choose one which offers you planned training, leading to nationally recognised qualifications.

Apprenticeships
If you want a job that combines training, and enables you to earn whilst you learn then an apprenticeship is the answer. More information can be found on www.apprenticeship.org.uk.

Entry to employment
If you're not ready to start an apprenticeship, employment with training or further education after Year 11, you may enrol on an Entry to Employment (e2e) programme. You must live in England and be aged between 16 and 18 years old. It will develop your motivation and confidence, allow you to try out different jobs, build your life skills and help you develop your Key Skills.

New Deal for Young People
New Deal is a government scheme designed to help people who are out of work. You'll be allocated an adviser who will help you to form a career and work plan. You can apply for the New Deal for Young People if you are aged between 18 and 24 years old and have had a continuous claim to Jobseekers' Allowance for six months or more. If you opt for

one of the full-time education or training options, your course fees will be paid. Help with the costs of books, travel or equipment is also available.

Study or training?
If your job offers little or no training, you may qualify for something called Time Off for Study or Training. You can qualify if you are 16 or 17 years old, and did not get any level 2 qualifications at school, which includes GCSEs at grades A*–C or an NVQ level 2.

Further information on funding, training, costs and options can be found at: www.jobcentreplus.gov.uk or www.learndirect.co.uk.

WHAT WILL I NEED TO PAY FOR?
When choosing a course you need to look carefully at what exactly you will have to pay for – not only in terms of the course itself but also the 'incidentals', such as travelling expenses and childcare. Expenses could include:

- registration fees
- specialist equipment (e.g. essential tools for beauty therapy)
- professional clothing (uniforms and shoes)
- general study materials, including photocopying, printing, computer disks and so on
- daily or weekly transport to college sites
- childcare
- travel to work placements, day visits or study tours
- general living expenses (accommodation, food and so on)
- fees for learning programmes (courses) and exam fees.

Although it is often difficult to meet all the costs of studying, it can be useful to find out any likely costs before you start a course. Some learning programmes or courses will be more expensive than others. Remember, you are entitled to ask for information about the costs of your particular course or programme, and colleges should provide written information and advice on fees, costs and student finance.

The costs can seem daunting, but don't panic! You should be able to get financial help with many of these things.

FINANCIAL HELP
The situation with regard to support and fees payment for part-time day or evening courses is more complicated:

- It's worth approaching the student awards department of your local authority (LA), who may be able to offer financial support for part-time students.
- If you're unemployed and claiming benefit you may still be able to study part time during the day up to a certain number of hours without it affecting your claim, under the New Deal programme. Check with your Jobcentre or benefits office.
- You may be able to get a Jobseeker's Allowance if you are studying part time.
- If you are working for an employer, there are training allowances available for employees.
- Once again, don't be shy about going to your local careers centre to find out more. Look at www.jobcentreplus.gov.uk.
- You may be eligible for an EMA (education maintenance allowance) during your study. Visit www.direct.gov.uk for more details.

Many part-time courses have reduced or concessionary fees. To be eligible, you must be in receipt of a means-tested benefit or be the unwaged dependant of someone who is receiving a benefit. To apply for fee reduction, you must enrol in person (or send photocopied details), so you can prove that you are genuinely entitled to reduced fees.

Spreading the cost
It may also be possible to pay in instalments for programmes costing more than £200 that are more than one term in length. A first payment of fees payable on enrolment and subsequent instalments over a few months is usual.

Travel
You may be entitled to help with travel costs if you apply to student services within a college. If not, it is possible to get some good deals on bus and train passes.

Examination fees
Students in receipt of a means-tested benefit or the unwaged dependant of someone in receipt of benefits can also get help with paying for examination fees. Ask your college guidance centre for details.

Loan advice
The college guidance centre can also help you with a Career Development Loan. This may sound a bit scary, but it could be a sensible option – think of it as investing in your future. Career Development Loans are a way of borrowing money to finance learning and have a special low interest rate. You can borrow anything from £300 to £8,000, which can be used to fund up to two years of learning plus up to one

year's practical work experience where it forms part of the course. The Learning and Skills Council (LSC) pays the interest on your loan while you're learning and for up to one month afterwards. You then repay the loan to the bank over an agreed period at a fixed rate of interest. For more information on Career Development Loans, ring 0800 585 505 or visit www.lifelonglearning.co.uk/cdl.

WHAT ABOUT CHILDCARE?

There may be some childcare places available at some colleges, but there are usually never enough, so speak to student services staff who may be able to help with suggestions. On some New Deal programmes, there may be funds available for childcare. Some other courses or learning programmes may also include an allowance for childcare, or you may be able to get some help from college learning support, access or welfare funds.

In some colleges or universities, you may be eligible for a small amount of money from the Access Fund or from any college welfare fund, learner support fund or hardship fund, if they exist at your place of study.

HELP AND GUIDANCE

You're probably thinking that there's a lot to take in here. There is, and it could well make sense to get further advice. Initially, it's probably best to ask staff at student services in the college. Do this as early as possible – **when you apply**. Don't wait until you enrol. Other sources of information and advice include your local Citizens Advice Bureau, welfare rights advisers in your local authority and your local library.

There's also an extensive list of resources in Chapter 9, which should provide you with many other leads.

CONGRATULATIONS – YOU'VE BEEN ACCEPTED!

Beauty therapy courses are vocational, which means that they are preparing you for the job that you will eventually do. So you need to remember that Industry Codes of Practice and conforming to regulations must start here. Your conduct, dress code and health and safety must be first rate. The job is providing a service to the public, and there is no room for sloppy service and couldn't-care-less attitudes.

You should consider a training centre as your employer. For example, don't be late for lessons and don't take sickies! Work as a team and respect your fellow students – this way you will be prepared for entry into a hard-working industry that thrives on its good reputation.

DID YOU KNOW?

Currently there are about 500 approved training providers offering beauty qualifications in the UK alone, both in further education colleges and in the private sector.

Now – imagine you've completed your course and you've graduated with flying colours. You've qualified, you're eager to get on with a real job in the beauty industry, you want to show the world what you're capable of. The next hurdle, then, is to find a job, and this is what we'll cover in the next chapter.

3

Job hunting for the beauty graduate

You've spotted an advertisement for your dream job, so what do you do next? In this chapter, we'll look at an overview of the process of applying for jobs and the interview process. For more detailed advice and information, you could also take a look at *Winning Interviews for First-time Job Hunters* and *Winning CVs for First-time Job Hunters* (2nd edition), both by Kath Houston, published by Trotman.

When job hunting, you will need to be organised. If you need to update your details, type out a letter of introduction or gather your certificates together, do this in good time. Job applications have closing dates, and if your application arrives just one day late, you will not get your chance to prove yourself. Your application will probably not even be looked at, even if you *really are* the perfect person for the job.

It is important that you make sure your CV and covering letter shines. Present yourself in your CV and covering letters as you will do in your professional life: immaculately and honestly.

Another possibility when job hunting is to use the services of a recruitment agency. See the box below and the list in Chapter 9 for more on recruitment companies specialising in the health and beauty industry.

RECRUITMENT COMPANIES
Recruitment companies specialise in matching the right candidate to the right job. Preparing your CV, writing the covering letter and developing your interview techniques are three of the most important stages in progressing your career, and they can advise you on this as well as help you find a job.

You need to register your details and current CV. This should always be free, and there is no obligation to accept the job that they match you with if, for example, something better comes along. Recruitment specialists should charge the company that they have managed to find an employee for rather than the employee themselves. They will want to interview you, too – and all the advice given below about interviews applies here as well.

CVs, LETTERS AND APPLICATION FORMS
CVs, covering letters and application forms are used in order to introduce yourself to the employer. Some jobs have hundreds of people applying for them so it's important that you stand out from the crowd. From the hundreds of job applications, just a few will be short-listed for an interview. Here are a few of the dos and don'ts when sending in an application for a job.

- Read the job advert very carefully – it's essential that you do exactly what the advert says. This may sound obvious, but it is surprising how many people ignore the instructions. For example, if an advert asks you to phone for further details in the first instance then do just that, don't send in your CV instead. All companies have their own format for recruitment, and if you get it wrong at first base what hope do you have of making a good impression?
- When putting together your CV, don't follow a model CV (for example, from a book or the Internet) slavishly. Make sure that you have added your own personal touch.
- One CV is not enough for a lifetime! Your education, work history and skills will develop over time, and it is essential that you update your CV yearly and that you also tailor it to each different job or purpose.
- In the beauty industry it is practical experience and good-quality college training that impress. Because salons and spas rely heavily on repeat bookings, they will be looking for candidates who don't have a history of moving about from job to job too regularly. Advertising the fact that you have worked in six different places in two years is not good!

If the company likes your covering letter, CV or application, they will select you for an interview. This is called short-listing.

INTERVIEWS

The interview could be with one person or with a panel of interviewers. The latter can be very daunting but, however many interviewers there are, you need to stay calm and look professional. It's about acting confidently and showing yourself in the best possible light.

In an interview panel for a beauty job, you might expect to find the manager (who wants to make sure that you would fit in with the team), perhaps the head therapist (who wants to ensure that your occupational standards and approach to client care are second to none and, in larger businesses, someone from human resources, which is responsible for the recruitment process.

Put aside time before the interview to find out a bit about the company and the job you are going for. Practise some typical interview questions and answers with a friend, and have ready a few of your own questions, such as 'Who will I report to?' or 'When will I know whether I have been selected?'. Practise the journey to the interview, time it and then still leave early on the day – just in case!

Before you set out, make sure that you have everything you need with you to prove that you have the right qualifications and experience – for example certificates or diplomas or a record of achievement if you are a school-leaver or student. If you are doing trade tests, you will also need to have your equipment, tools and uniform (more on this below).

The most important things to remember for an interview are:

- smile and be friendly
- be yourself and never pretend to be someone you are not; it will be hard to live up to if you are selected
- maintain good posture when walking into the room and sitting down
- use positive body language with good eye contact
- sit only when invited to and don't slouch in the seat

- don't smoke (even beforehand – your clothes will smell) or chew gum
- personal hygiene is important, make sure you are freshly showered and your breath is fresh.

Appearance is crucial in an interview for a job in the beauty industry. Remember that you will be almost a walking advert for the company's services or products. You need to:

- wear smart, clean, ironed clothes and polished shoes
- if you wear make-up, make sure it is well-applied; it definitely should not be heavy
- make sure your nails are well manicured and fairly short; having long/artificial nails when being interviewed for a job as a beauty therapist will be a real turn-off for employers
- make sure your hair is neat, clean and free from split ends or roots growing out.

When answering questions, always have the evidence ready to back up your statements and claims. If, for example, the interviewer asks you whether you are good at working in a team, make sure you can back this up with an instance where you have shown this – whether in a job or at college or somewhere else.

If you get to the interview stage but are unsuccessful, make sure you ask for feedback as to why you were not selected.

Here are a few good examples of strengths and weaknesses to identify in interview (remember, always be ready to give an example of where you have shown any strengths that you mention):

- good timekeeping
- ability to get on with people and work as a team
- professional attitude
- organisational skills.

Some weaknesses:

- a bit of a perfectionist, like everything to be in order
- spending too much money on clothes and beauty magazines.

These weaknesses could turn to your advantage and be looked on as strengths, because they show that you like things to be organised and just right; also that you keep up-to-date with beauty and fashion.

TRADE TESTS

Because beauty therapy is a practical occupation, part of the interview process will include what is known as a 'trade test' or 'skills test'. This is when you will be asked to demonstrate a practical treatment on someone so that the company can view your practical skills and techniques. This is often done at a second interview after the company has first seen you, talked to you and felt that you could fit in as part of the team.

Trade tests can be a very nerve-racking experience, but don't worry – interviewers will usually take nerves into

Immaculate appearance and hygiene are essential during a trade test.

consideration in their assessment of you. Some employers will let you know beforehand which treatments you will be expected to carry out on the day. This is a much fairer system as it allows you time to prepare, which in turn will help to calm your nerves.

Again, immaculate appearance and hygiene are essential during a trade test. You should wear clean and ironed clothes, along with clean, sensible shoes. Long hair should be tied back neatly without any wispy stray hairs. Any make-up should be subtle and not caked on! Nails should be natural, short and without nail varnish, unless you are applying for a job as a nail technician. All jewellery including your watch should be removed.

There really is no excuse for a sloppy appearance. If you fail to do any of the above, you simply will not be offered the job.

From a professional point of view, there are a few things you must do during a trade test. It's easy to forget the simplest tasks when you are nervous, so familiarise yourself with the treatment basics.

- Prepare your work area with all the cotton wool, tissues, towels, products and equipment that you will need, including a disinfectant solution for sanitising tools and a record card.
- Meet and greet the client with a big smile and friendly approach.

- Introduce yourself!
- Make a quick check of the client's medical history to ensure that they are suitable for treatment (even if a member of staff in the salon) and enter it onto a record card.
- Prepare the client by giving them a gown and showing them to the couch or chair – help them onto the couch.
- If a gown is not available or suitable for the treatment, protect clothing with a towel and couch roll.
- Ask if the client is comfortable and warm.
- Explain that you are going to wash your hands before you start.
- Explain what you are about to do before starting the treatment.
- Carry out the treatment with care and attention to detail.
- Check occasionally that the client is still comfortable.
- Keep your work area tidy throughout the treatment by throwing away waste immediately in a bin next to the work area and by replacing bottle tops straight away.
- Don't use your couch as a trolley top; this only shows bad habits and could result in spillage or accidents.
- When you have finished, help the client off the couch, ask if they enjoyed it and, most importantly, thank them for their time.
- Wash your hands and return to your assessor for feedback.
- Hope for the best!

TELEPHONE INTERVIEWS

Interviews by phone are becoming more popular with some employers in the hair and beauty industries. They are used as a first interview and can save valuable time for the company. If the employer likes the sound of you on the telephone, then you will be asked to attend a face-to-face interview. As with all interviews, preparation and organisation is the key. Don't ever get casual in your approach to job hunting.

You won't remember everything, so have your CV, application form, covering letter and the job advert out in front of you before the call. It's a good idea to stand up when you are speaking; surprisingly enough, you will sound more businesslike and less casual than if you are slouching on a chair. Try to sound cheerful, enthusiastic and interested, and avoid using slang such as 'OK', 'yeah' or 'right'. For more advice about telephone interviews, see *Winning Interviews for First-time Job Hunters*.

THE JOB OFFER

If you get to the interview stage but are unsuccessful, most companies are quite happy to give you feedback as to why you were not selected. This is helpful when applying for your next position. Learn by your experiences!

If, on the other hand, the company decides that you are the best person for the job, they will offer you the job – having first checked your references, of course. They may telephone you first and, if you accept, they will send you a formal letter outlining the offer. This will detail the terms and

Being asked what your weaknesses are is always a difficult question to answer because you can easily land yourself in it. Prepare an answer beforehand.

conditions – for example, what you will be paid, your hours of work, your holiday entitlement and so on. You need to check these out carefully before writing a formal letter of acceptance. Talk to the appropriate person on the telephone if you need anything clarified.

If you are not entirely satisfied with the terms and conditions of the job offer you may be in a position to negotiate, especially if you have a wealth of experience and technical skills (a newly qualified therapist, though, is not really in a position to negotiate). If this is the case, write a letter thanking the company for the offer of a job, explain that you are very keen to work with them but would like to know whether their formal offer terms are negotiable. Whatever aspect – pay, hours, holiday and so on – you would like improved upon, state this in the letter. Also explain that you will contact them within a day or two with a follow-up telephone call to discuss this further. They will then be in no doubt that you are still keen on the job. However, bear in mind that negotiating a better deal can be risky and could cost you a job that you would have taken anyway.

When you finally accept a job, you and the company will enter a contract of employment, which details the terms and conditions you have agreed upon. It is a legal requirement for employers to give you this in writing within two months of starting work for them.

Quite often the job will be offered on a trial period for a few months to check that you are suitable for the job. After this probationary time, if you have proved yourself, the job will become permanent.

Of course, you may decide to turn down the offer. Again, politeness and manners are the key – never alienate an employer as you may come across them later on in your career.

In the next chapter, we'll look more closely at the issue of pay. It can be a thorny issue in the beauty industry, and you need to be aware of your rights.

Pay and perks

4

Traditionally, people working in the beauty industry were very poorly paid – something that helps explain the massive shortage of qualified workers today. However, things are changing and while starting salaries may still seem low, there are plenty of opportunities for much bigger salaries in the industry. Some typical annual incomes might be:

- starting salaries for beauty therapists are around £10,000–£15,000 a year
- experienced therapists can earn between £15,000 and £20,000 a year
- salon managers can earn over £20,000 a year.

These figures are only a guideline; they vary depending on area, size of business and individual responsibilities.

There are likely to be regional variations in salaries for some positions. For example, working in a Central London salon, possibly with high-profile clients, you could earn substantially more than the figures indicated above. Salaries can also include an addition to the basic pay called London weighting, awarded because the cost of living in London is so high. Other parts of the UK are expensive to live and work in too, so ideally a salary ought to make an allowance for this. However, only when you have reached a senior position can you expect to benefit from regionally enhanced pay. This is why many graduates tend to work locally at first in order to gain much needed experience rather than travel to other parts of the country.

The minimum wage is a legal right which covers almost all workers above compulsory school leaving age. It came into force on 1 April 1999 and since then it has ensured that employees have some protection against poor salaries. There are different minimum wage rates for different groups of workers; the most common are listed below.

- The main rate for workers aged 22 and over increased on 1 October 2006 to £5.35 an hour from £5.05 an hour
- The development rate (for people on training and development programmes of study) for 18–21 year olds increased to £4.45 an hour from £4.25 an hour
- The development rate for 16–17 year olds increased to £3.30 an hour from £3.00 an hour.

The amount rises yearly and from 1 October 2007 the minimum wage will increase again as follows:

- adult rate (workers aged 22 and over) will increase to £5.52
- development rate for 18-21 year olds will increase to £4.60
- development rate for 16-17 year olds will increase to £3.40.

Minimum wages for government-funded schemes and apprenticeships may differ; full details on all wage mimimums can be found on www.direct.gov.uk and www.berr.gov.uk.

PERKS OF THE JOB

A job in the beauty industry has always provided a bonus – the chance to be pampered yourself! After all, it's just as important that you look as well-groomed and relaxed as your clients. If there is a gap in the appointments column and there are no other jobs to be done, then it is accepted practice that staff carry out treatments or practise new skills on each other – as long as it doesn't affect their work.

A job in the beauty industry has always provided a bonus – the chance to be pampered yourself!

It would never be acceptable, however, to book staff treatments in an appointment column at the expense of a paying client. Each company will have their own policy on staff treatments, and it is important that you check this beforehand. It may be, for instance, that the company asks its staff to make a small contribution towards the products used in the treatment.

Other incentives on offer in some companies include commission payments based on your sales and occasionally your sales and treatments. This is particularly likely to be the case if you are a productive therapist who brings in a good profit for them – they will want to keep you as an employee and not lose you to another company. Commission can typically be 10% of your takings (or more in some parts of the UK or in retailing jobs), so this can certainly boost your weekly wage.

DID YOU KNOW?

The average number of clients visiting a small salon per week is 125 and for a large salon 26

A further perk is the tips. This is a very common occurrence in beauty-therapy establishments when clients are pleased with the treatment and service they have received.

This begs the question, of course – what exactly does make for excellent service and a professional treatment in the beauty industry? You'll have picked up many of the main points already, but in the next chapter we'll look more closely at the special qualities that go into the making of a truly excellent beauty specialist or therapist.

5

Tools of the trade

Academic skills are important, but what makes a good, as opposed to a merely competent, beauty therapist are a few special attributes and qualities, many of which can be summed up as **people skills** – the ability to interact with all types of people from all walks of life regardless of age, ethnicity, gender or personality.

THE MUST-HAVES

Being able to **make clients feel at ease** helps make sure they will rebook. Awkward silences and stilted conversations can make people feel embarrassed and self-conscious, especially when the type of treatment being carried out is of a very personal nature.

Some people are 'naturals' – they find it easy to talk to clients and are easy to warm to. Others find it harder, but many of these qualities will come with practice and experience. The most important personality qualities are:

● **good communication skills** – you must be good at explaining treatments and how products work

DID YOU KNOW?

A small salon retains a higher percentage of clients than a large one. Is this perhaps due to better — that is, more personal — customer care?

- **organisational skills** – there can be a lot of filing and paperwork as well as computer record systems
- **a smart appearance and good hygiene**
- **a friendly and welcoming manner** that puts clients at ease
- **patience and good listening skills**
- **a positive attitude** – you have to show confidence and belief in the treatments and products you are offering
- **a caring and respectful manner**
- **stamina and strength** – you will be on your feet all day and some treatments (for example massage) are very strenuous
- **strong hands**
- **an ability to show calmness** when everything around you seems manic – a hectic or panic-stricken reaction when it's busy or when things don't go quite to plan will do nothing to reassure your client
- **good health and a high level of fitness**
- **artistic flair** – for example for nail art and make-up
- **knowledge of anatomy, physiology and chemistry** or at least an aptitude to learn
- **commercial ability** – for example, being able to work to recommended timescales for profit and commission
- **an ability to sell and promote** products and treatments to clients.

Beauty therapy is a caring profession, so make sure that your actions and thoughts towards others reflect this.

One other big quality needed when working in a salon, big or small, is the **ability to work as a team** and get on with a wide range of colleagues. This doesn't mean that you need to be best friends with everyone, but what it does mean is that you will be expected to give and take – to be civil, friendly and cooperative.

One other big quality needed when working in a salon, big or small, is the ability to work as a team.

THE 'DEFINITELY NOTS'

There are some things that you won't be able to do much about but which will make a career in beauty therapy a bad choice. These might include medical reasons such as a bad back or allergies to lots of cosmetic products.

Bad attitude is something you can do something about, although some people refuse to believe that they are the ones with the problem! If you can't be bothered to put yourself out and always give the best that you can, then start looking for an alternative career now. Beauty therapy is a caring profession, so make sure that your actions and thoughts towards others reflect this. A short temper and unhelpful attitude are the last things needed in a busy salon. Clients can be demanding – and rightly so. They are paying money to be pampered and to receive a high standard of treatment.

6

Treatments of the trade

If you're reading this book, you are clearly interested in taking up a career in beauty therapy, but how much of an idea do you really have of what it's all about? You may have had a few treatments yourself as a client, or you may even have done a few treatments for friends or neighbours on a casual basis, but many people are still surprised at just how involved beauty treatment is. It's not just a case of applying make-up or waxing a person's legs!

As well as the close personal contact, you will also be expected to operate mechanical and electrical machines as part of a treatment, have extensive knowledge of the muscles and bones and learn the science behind the treatments. In the box on the next page, you'll find a brief explanation of the main beauty treatments available in the UK today.

It is essential that you have extensive insurance cover and abide by the rules and guidelines of the insurance policy in order to remain covered.

Many of the treatments listed are complex – and very occasionally things can go wrong. This is why all beauty specialists and therapists must have insurance. Insurance is not just a safety net in case you cause injury or damage to a client or her belongings; it is also there to protect you as a therapist. Unfortunately in today's world, people are making insurance claims against companies far more frequently than ever before so it is essential that you have extensive cover and abide by the rules and guidelines of the insurance policy in order to remain covered.

These are just a few of the most well known treatments. Carry out some research on other holistic and beauty treatments — you'll be surprised how many there are.

A–Z OF BEAUTY TREATMENTS
If you think you want to be a beauty therapist make sure you know what treatments you may be expected to carry out.

Aromatherapy – Essential oils extracted from plant and herb sources are used through massage to alleviate a wide variety of conditions, to relieve stress and induce relaxation.

Electrical body treatments – A range of electrical equipment is used to achieve better muscle and skin tone. Some treatments can aid slimming and improve the appearance of cellulite.

Electrical epilation – The removal of unwanted hair through the application of a low-level electrical current. Eventually the treatment can permanently destroy the hair.

Electrical face treatments – A range of electrical equipment is used to achieve better muscle and skin tone as well as for deep cleansing and anti-wrinkle treatments.

Eye treatments – This could include: eyelash tinting to darken lashes, eyebrow shaping to enhance the shape of the brow and eyebrow tinting to darken pale or grey brows. False lashes can also be applied to increase the length and thickness of the lashes.

Fake (self) tanning – This is tanning the safe way. The therapist applies a temporary tanning lotion to your body to deepen your natural skin tone. This is applied with the hands or sprayed on and lasts for about a week.

Heat and bath treatments – Hydrotherapy (water therapy) can be very effective in relieving stress, aches and pains and as a preheating treatment prior to massage. Spa treatments are spa, steam and sauna.

Indian head massage – Also known as *champissage*, this is an ancient technique which involves massaging and rubbing the head, neck and shoulders. It is used for stress relief.

Lash perming – This enhances the lashes by temporarily curling them.

Make-up – Products used to enhance the natural appearance of the skin and facial features. Make-up effects can be for day or evening; they can be corrective, dramatic, theatrical, photographic and so on.

Manicures and pedicures – This involves treatment on skin of the hands and feet, the nails and the surrounding cuticles. Products are used to massage, remove dead dry skin, soften, shape and polish.

Manual body massage – Usually Swedish massage. Movements are used to improve the blood flow, exercise the muscles and relax the body. Hands are used for flowing movements, such as stroking, friction movements, such as kneading, and stimulating movements, such as beating and cupping.

Manual facial – This treatment deep-cleans the skin, exfoliates dead skin cells and removes blackheads; it also includes a massage of the face, neck and shoulders and a face mask. No electrical equipment is used, it is all hands-on.

Nail techniques – This involves applying extensions to the natural nail with gel or acrylic; it also includes nail art.

Reflexology – This consists of pressure massage on the reflex points of the hands or feet. These reflex points mirror the body. The treatment unblocks the energy lines to aid self-healing and body rebalancing.

Ultraviolet (UV) tanning – This is tanning of the skin by application of UV rays from a sunbed or solarium. This must be closely monitored by experienced staff so as not to permanently damage the skin.

Wax depilation – This is the removal of unwanted hair, usually on the legs, underarm, bikini and facial area. *Warm wax* is thinly applied to the skin. The wax sticks to the hairs, which enables them and their follicles to be removed when a paper or fabric strip is applied and pulled off again. *Hot wax* is applied thickly with a spatula and flicked off with the fingers.

With the increase in more specialised treatments, such as laser, semi-permanent make-up and electrical treatments, there is more reason than ever to ensure good training that is industry recognised in order to get treatment liability cover.

It takes a very long time to develop even a part of all the skills and knowledge needed in the beauty industry. Good basic training is a must, of course – but no one in this business really ever stops learning. In the following chapter, we'll look at what training actually involves and how you can continue to train and learn throughout your career.

7

Training

As we have already seen, training plays a crucial role in the beauty industry. In this chapter, we will look a little more carefully at each stage of the training process – from initial training at entry level into the profession to ongoing career development.

There is a wide range of courses and qualifications in the UK. It depends on different factors as to which method of training you choose – if you learn best by being continually assessed, then an NVQ/SVQ might be your best option; if you prefer to sit final examinations, then there are courses that offer this. We'll cover both these options below.

Training at private centres is usually shorter and more intensive than in further education colleges and with smaller class sizes. However, private centres may not be approved to offer nationally recognised qualifications and could have their own certificates of achievement. Take care – these are not always recognised as a valid qualification by employers. You must check what qualification you will get at the end of the private course because it may also be difficult to get insurance (see Chapter 6 for more on insurance). ITEC, NVQ and VTCT courses tend to be studied at a college or adult education centre, while CIDESCO and CIBTAC tend to be offered at private training establishments and as such can be expensive.

NVQ1 → **BEAUTY THERAPY OR RECEPTION ASSISTANT**

SALONS, SPAS, HEALTH CLUBS

NVQ2 → **BEAUTY SPECIALIST**

CHOICE OF GENERAL, MAKE-UP OR NAIL SERVICES ROUTE

SALONS, MOBILE, NAIL BARS
OR RENT-A-CHAIR, COSMETIC COUNTERS

NVQ3 → **BEAUTY THERAPIST**

CHOICE OF GENERAL, MAKE-UP, NAIL SERVICES OR SPA THERAPY ROUTE

SALONS, SPAS, SALON OWNER, THEATRE, TELEVISION, HOSPITALS, COMPLEMENTARY THERAPY CENTRES, ELECTROLYSIS CLINICS, HEALTH CLUBS, HEALTH FARMS, TRAINING CENTRES

THE NVQ/SVQ ROUTE

The Hairdressing and Beauty Industry Authority (Habia) states that there are no recommended formal entry requirements for acceptance into training for NVQ/SVQ levels 1 and 2 and that the industry is more attracted by the qualities that a trainee has to offer. So, although some colleges do ask for GCSEs in Maths and English as a minimum entry requirement, learners are often judged on their individual merits even if they have not reached the required academic level to be accepted on a course.

NVQ/SVQs are made up of units and have a structure a little like building-blocks that build up to a complete qualification. There are strict criteria that a student must meet at every unit and every level in order for him or her to be judged competent at a particular skill. There are mandatory and optional units. Mandatory units cover the essential areas of the job and must be taken to pass the whole qualification, whereas optional units can be chosen to suit the student's own needs and preferences. Additional help in the form of learning support is available in further education colleges, so if you struggle with paperwork, can't get organised or have difficulty understanding some of the terminology or

Additional help in the form of learning support is available in further education colleges, so if you struggle with paperwork, can't get organised or have difficulty understanding some of the terminology or assignments, accept the help on offer in order to pass your course.

assignments, accept the help on offer in order to pass your course.

NVQs are work-related, competence-based qualifications. Completion of an NVQ shows that you can actually do the job and not just talk about it! NVQs reflect the skills and expertise needed to do a job well.

Standards are developed by standards setting bodies or National Training Organisations (NTOs). The standards in Hairdressing and Beauty Therapy are set by Habia.

These standards are mainly employer and industry led. In other words, employers tell the setting bodies:

● what they expect trainees to be learning in order to be successful in a job
● what they need to know and the skills they need to be able to demonstrate
● what they expect from their employees once in the salon.

Assessment for NVQ/SVQs is continuous throughout training and therefore avoids the need for a final examination. Assessment is carried out using various methods, including practical observation, written tasks and assignments and case studies. You'll also be expected to:

● compile a portfolio of evidence
● practise all skills on fellow students
● carry out practical treatment assessments on clients
● sit end-of-unit tests.

Each practical skill must be assessed as competent in a **realistic working environment** and on a 'real client' in order for the student to be awarded that skill.

There is no set time limit for completion of an NVQ/SVQ, but after you have enrolled on a course you will be registered with the college and an awarding body. This registration will usually last up to three years, but if you take longer you will need to re-register and pay an additional fee along with extra tuition fees if requested by the college or centre. However qualification structures change regularly and if you take too long to complete one you may need to start again as your skills will not be classed as current. At a college of further education the average length of training on a full-time basis is one year for level 2 and two years to gain up to level 3.

At present there is not a complete level 4 structure for beauty therapy but there are individual qualifications available at level 4 standard designed specifically for continuing professional development. Level 4 units generally include organising staff in work and training, maintaining the financial side, business planning and keeping everything running smoothly – from the stock to the appointments!

THE EXAMINATION ROUTE

Awarding bodies that offer the examination route are CIBTAC/ CIDESCO and ITEC. If you follow this route, you will be expected to study for a set amount of hours laid down by the awarding body. At the end of the course, every student must sit a theory examination as well as a practical examination for each subject learnt. Check out the CIBTAC/CIDESCO and ITEC websites for more information about the content of both courses and what you need to do to pass.

NVQ/SVQ Apprenticeships

These are work-based learning programmes aimed at young people from the age of 16. An apprentice earns whilst learning on a government recognised course. Apprentices are employees of the salon in which they work. They attend training one day a week, which includes the technical skills and Key Skills. At the end of the apprenticeship you could be qualified to work in hairdressing, beauty therapy, nails services, spa therapy or barbering. To find out more, contact your local Learning and Skills Council (LSC) or careers office or visit www.apprenticeship.org.uk.

Diplomas

These are very new and exciting qualifications which are being introduced into schools from September 2007. The idea is that every young person in a school or college should be entitled to follow any one of the diploma courses at an appropriate level for them, wherever they are in the country. This entitlement will be in place by 2013, once all of the diplomas have been tested. There are 14 subject areas which are being phased in. Hair and beauty therapy is scheduled for September 2009.

Students will be able to select which level diploma suits them best.

- Level 1: equivalent to 4–5 GCSEs at grades D to G
- Level 2: equivalent to 5–6 GCSEs at grades A* to C
- Level 3: equivalent to three A-levels.

A diploma is an all-round package which gives students the right knowledge, experience, insight and attitude to prepare them for the next stage in life – whether that's university, college or work. It is recognised that not all students will follow an academic route of study at school; there are many pupils that are much more suited to the vocational route.

FURTHER TRAINING AND CONTINUING PROFESSIONAL DEVELOPMENT (CPD)

Although there are some excellent basic qualification courses available out there, no one can learn everything at college. Once you've achieved your beauty therapy qualification you will need to continue your learning. A lot, of course, can be learnt through experience and years in practice, but additional and ongoing training will help to refresh, deepen and extend a therapist's knowledge and understanding. You may also want to train further in order to specialise.

This is especially true in industries like hairdressing and beauty therapy, where new techniques, products and equipment mean constant updating is essential for consistent and improving standards. Beauty therapy is a rapidly changing industry – practitioners need to keep up to date with the latest techniques and information and to continue the process of 'life-long learning'.

Indeed, ongoing training may eventually become compulsory for all beauty and holistic therapists. Until recently the abbreviation CPD – Continuing Professional Development – was familiar only to therapists working in education and nursing, where normally a certain number of hours of ongoing learning are required in order to keep your job. But this is no longer the case. It is now considered good practice for everyone to develop and increase their skills on a regular basis. At the moment it is only essential for teachers and assessors of hair and beauty to do this. If beauty and complementary therapy is finally regulated, it is likely that everyone will need to show evidence of continuing education. However, there is no reason for anyone to wait until this becomes compulsory. Start now and be ahead of the game. Here are a few tips to help you.

Attendance at trade events, seminars and workshops will also count toward your Continuing Professional Development hours.

- Spend every possible moment to develop your knowledge and practise your skills. Don't relax just because you have a qualification. Read every book, magazine and trade journal (see the lists in Chapter 9) you can lay your hands on to get the latest beauty buzzword on everyone's lips. Clients expect you to know about what they might have read in an article – they look to you as the expert in the field of beauty.
- Attend trade shows and exhibitions (see Chapter 9) and workshops for professional development; never think you know it all just because you have qualified – you don't. Join professional organisations (see Chapter 9) to keep you informed about new developments and in contact with other therapists with whom you can share knowledge and advice.
- CPD in the industry is good practice. It will set you apart from the complacent comfortable existence of those who sit back and expect jobs and business to fall into their laps!
- Enrol on your next course now! Map out a five-year learning plan to extend your talents and flair and get a head start.

8

The last word

Your head is now crammed with information and training options for beauty therapy. This book should have given you an insight into the industry so that now you can choose the career path that's right for you whether you are a new trainee or graduate. You now need to make the plunge – making the major decisions that will get you on the road to qualifications… and success!

The future looks bright if you:

- train in the basics first – there are no short cuts if you want your appointment columns full
- listen to your educators (that is, your college lecturers, trainers, assessors and employers) – together they have years of experience and will be ready with a wise word every now and then
- hear what people have to say and learn from them; don't get set in your ways – the industry develops and moves forward rapidly
- develop new skills and ideas continually
- teach others 'good practice' by example
- always strive to be the best you can.

Finally, good luck!

If you have made it this far through the book then you should know if the **beauty industry** really is the career for you. But before contacting the professional bodies listed in the next chapter, here's a final, fun checklist to show if you have chosen wisely.

THE LAST WORD ✔ TICK YES OR NO

DO YOU LIKE WORKING WITH YOUR HANDS?
- ☐ YES
- ☐ NO

DO YOU LIKE WORKING CLOSELY WITH OTHER PEOPLE?
- ☐ YES
- ☐ NO

DO YOU CONSIDER YOURSELF TO BE FIT AND HEALTHY WITH GOOD STAMINA?
- ☐ YES
- ☐ NO

ARE YOU SELF MOTIVATED AND ABLE TO THINK ON YOUR FEET?
- ☐ YES
- ☐ NO

DO YOU WANT TO DO A JOB THAT MAKES PEOPLE FEEL GOOD ABOUT THEMSELVES?
- ☐ YES
- ☐ NO

DO YOU WANT TO SEE THE WORLD?
- ☐ YES
- ☐ NO

ARE YOU MOTIVATED TO LEARN NEW SKILLS?
- ☐ YES
- ☐ NO

If you answered 'YES' to all these questions then
CONGRATULATIONS! YOU'VE CHOSEN THE RIGHT CAREER
If you answered 'NO' to any of these questions then this may not be the career for you.

Further information

9

In this chapter you will find contact information for the relevant government and industry advisory, training, awarding and professional bodies for the beauty industry as well as further sources of information in the way of books, trade journals and websites. There is a wealth of information and advice out there – explore!

AWARDING BODIES

These are the organisations that provide recognised qualifications within the beauty industry.

City & Guilds

1 Giltspur Street
London
EC1A 9DD
020 7294 2800
www.city-and-guilds.co.uk

Comité International d'Estéthique et de Cosmétologie (CIDESCO)

Waidstrasse 4a
8037 Zürich
Switzerland
00 41 44 448 2200
www.cidesco.com

Confederation of International Beauty Therapy and Cosmetology (CIBTAC)
Meteor Court
Barnett Way
Gloucester
GL4 3GG
01452 623114
www.cibtac.com

Edexcel
One90 High Holborn
London
WC1V 7BH
0870 240 9800
www.edexcel.org.uk

ITEC
2nd Floor, Chiswick Gate
598–608 Chiswick High Road
London
W4 5RT
020 8994 4141
www.itecworld.co.uk

Vocational Training and Charitable Trust (VTCT)
3rd Floor, Eastleigh House
Upper Market Street
Eastleigh
Hampshire
SO50 9FD
www.vtct.org.uk

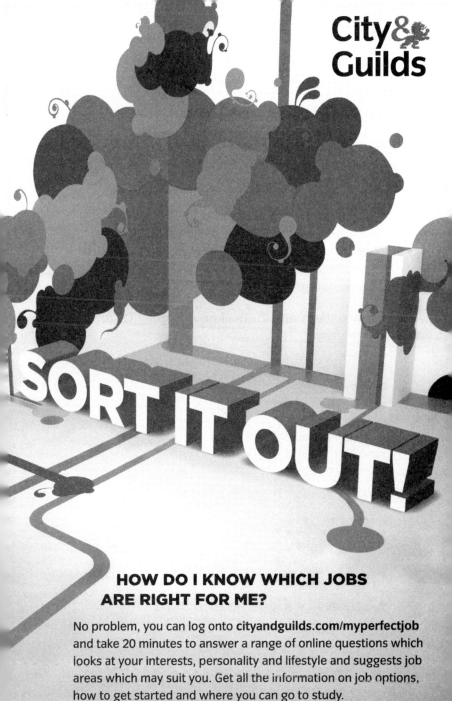

City& Guilds

SORT IT OUT!

HOW DO I KNOW WHICH JOBS ARE RIGHT FOR ME?

No problem, you can log onto **cityandguilds.com/myperfectjob** and take 20 minutes to answer a range of online questions which looks at your interests, personality and lifestyle and suggests job areas which may suit you. Get all the information on job options, how to get started and where you can go to study.
cityandguilds.com/myperfectjob

QUALIFICATION REGULATORY BODIES

Hairdressing and Beauty Industry Authority (Habia)
Oxford House
Sixth Avenue
Sky Business Park
Robin Hood Airport
Doncaster
DN9 3GG
0845 230 6080
www.habia.org

Qualifications and Curriculum Authority (QCA)
83 Piccadilly
London
W1J 8QA
020 7509 5555
www.qca.org.uk

Scottish Qualifications Authority (SQA)
The Optima Building
58 Robertson Street
Glasgow
G2 8DQ
0845 279 1000
www.sqa.org.uk

PROFESSIONAL MEMBERSHIP BODIES

Association of Nail Technicians (ANT)
16 Bourne Road
Bexley
Kent
DA5 1LU
01322 555724
www.ant.uk.net

Association of Reflexologists (AOR)
5 Fore Street
Taunton
Somerset
TA1 1HX
0870 567 3320
www.aor.org.uk

British Association of Beauty Therapy and Cosmetology (BABTAC)
Ambrose House
Meteor Court
Barnett Way
Barnwood
Gloucester
GL4 3GG
0845 065 9000
www.babtac.com

British Association of Electrolysists (BAE)
40 Parkfield Road
Ickenham
Middlesex
UB10 8LW
0870 128 0477
www.electrolysis.co.uk

British Federation of Massage Practitioners (BFMP)
78 Meadow Street
Preston
PR1 1TS
01772 881063
www.jolanta.co.uk

The British Reflexology Association (BRA)
Administration Office
Monks Orchard
Whitbourne
Worcester
WR6 5RB
01886 821207
www.britreflex.co.uk

Federation of Holistic Therapists (FHT)
18 Shakespeare Business Centre
Hathaway Close
Eastleigh
Hampshire
SO50 4SR
0870 420 2022
www.fht.org.uk

Freelance Hair and Beauty Federation (FHBF)
01582 431783
www.fhbf.org.uk

General Council for Massage Therapy (GCMT)
27 Old Gloucester Street
London
WC1N 3XX
0870 850 4452
www.gcmt.org.uk

The Guild of Professional Beauty Therapists (GPBT)
Guild House
320 Burton Road
Derby